American College of Surgeons
Protocol for Cancer Surgery Documentation: Thyroid Cancer

Name: ACS.CSSP.protocol.thyroid.2023.v1

What This Protocol Includes and Covers

- A synoptic operative report for thyroid cancer surgery
    - Section 1: EMR Autopopulated Information
    - Section 2: Tumor-Specific Information (required)
    - Section 3: Additional Procedure Details
- The synoptic operative report summary template
- Knowledge Platform with explanatory notes

American College of Surgeons Standards References

The following ACS standards references are heavily leveraged throughout the synoptic operative report and Knowledge Platform: *AJCC Cancer Staging Manual, Eighth Edition; Operative Standards for Cancer Surgery,* Volume 2; and *Standards for Oncology Registry Entry (STORE) 2023.*

Authors

Tracy S. Wang, MD, FACS*; Elizabeth G. Grubbs, MD, MS, FACS*; Julie F. McGill, MD, FACS*; Carmen C. Solorzano, MD, FACS*; Cord Sturgeon, MD, MS, FACS*

Reviewers

Christopher E. Fundakowski, MD, FACS†; Kepal N. Patel, MD, FACS†; Terry Sarantou, MD, FACS†

Contributors

Peter Angelos, MD, PhD, FACS; Sylvia L. Asa, MD, PhD; Denise Carneiro-Pla, MD, FACS; Herbert Chen, MD, FACS; Douglas B. Evans, MD, FACS; Raymon Grogan, MD, MS, FACS; David T. Hughes, MD, FACS; Carrie C. Lubitz, MD, FACS; Jennifer E. Rosen, MD, FACS; David F. Schneider, MD, MS, FACS; Wen Shen, MD, MA, FACS; Julie Ann Sosa, MD, MA, FACS; R. Michael Tuttle, MD; Linwah Yip, MD, FACS; Mark Zafereo, MD, FACS

**Denotes primary author. †Denotes synoptic operative report reviewer.*

Synoptic Operative Report

What This Synoptic Operative Report Includes and Covers
This synoptic operative report (SOR) covers thyroid cancer surgery documentation.

The SOR includes roughly 15 fields for EMR autopopulated data, 10 fields for tumor-specific data *(required)*, and 8 fields for additional procedure data that assist with billing and regulatory and practice requirements. This synoptic operative report was designed for cases of primary thyroid malignancy or thyroid neoplasms, and not for benign disease. However, narrative text boxes may facilitate expanded use of this synoptic report at the user's discretion.

How Tthis Synoptic Operative Report Is Organized
Required fields are indicated by an asterisk (*).

Section 1: EMR Autopopulated Information

Patient Name*
Patient ID*
Date of Surgery*
Name of Surgeon*
Name of Co-Surgeon
Name of Assistant(s)
Indication for Surgery*
Preoperative Diagnosis*
Postoperative Diagnosis*
Procedure(s) Performed*
Specimens Removed
Type of Anesthesia
Estimated Blood Loss
Drain/Implant
Additional Administrative Details

Section 2: Tumor-Specific Information *(required)*

Number of Foci*
Preoperative Biopsy Performed*
Molecular Testing Performed on Biopsy*
Clinical Nodal Status*
Procedure Performed*
Intent of Surgery*
Macroscopic Disease Status of Primary Tumor*
Central Compartment Lymph Node Dissection*
Lateral Compartment Lymph Node Dissection*
Macroscopic Completeness of Resection*

Section 3: Additional Procedure Details

Neuromonitoring Used
Recurrent Laryngeal Nerve(s)
External Branch of the Superior Laryngeal Nerve(s)
Parathyroid Glands
Pyramidal Lobe
Operative Approach
Additional Surgical Information
Intraoperative Complications

Instructions

This report is intended for documentation at the completion of each surgical procedure.

Instructions are provided for each data field.

Explanatory notes provide reference material for each data field.

Narrative boxes are available in all sections of the SOR to allow the addition of provider-specific information as needed.

Completing all applicable data fields in the SOR will generate a SOR summary that is compliant with multiple regulatory requirements.

- **Section 1 Instructions:** You are being asked to review all the data fields in Section 1 as the information is autopopulated from the EMR and should be checked for accuracy. Please make corrections as needed and be sure to complete required fields. Throughout the tool, required fields are marked with an asterisk (*) and represent best practice.
- **Section 2 Instructions:** You are asked to complete all data fields in this section (Tumor-Specific Information) because they are required as best practice.
- **Section 3 Instructions:** You are not required to complete these data fields, but the additional surgical data elements included in this section (Additional Procedure Details) will support diverse coding, regulatory, and practice needs.

Section 1: EMR Autopopulated Information (Note A)

Patient Name*
Patient ID*
Date of Surgery*
Name of Surgeon*
Name of Co-Surgeon
Name of Assistant(s)
Indication for Surgery*
Preoperative Diagnosis*
Postoperative Diagnosis*
Procedure(s) Performed*
Specimens Removed
Type of Anesthesia
Estimated Blood Loss
Drain/Implant
Additional Administrative Details

Section 2: Tumor-Specific Information (Note B)

Preoperative Assessment

*** Number of Foci** (Note C)
Select single best answer.
__ Unifocal disease
[If "Unifocal disease" is selected, display the following:]
*** Tumor Location** (Note D)
Select single best answer.
__ Right lobe
__ Left lobe
__ Isthmus
__ Pyramidal lobe
__ Unknown/Other [*Narrative Box*]

*** Tumor Size** (Note E)
Round to the nearest tenth of a centimeter.
__._ cm

*** Evidence of Extrathyroidal Extension of Tumor on Imaging** (Note F)
Select single best answer.
__ No
__ Yes

__ Multifocal disease
[If "Multifocal disease" is selected, display the following:]
*** Primary Tumor Location** (Note D)
Select single best answer.
__ Right lobe
__ Left lobe
__ Isthmus
__ Pyramidal lobe
__ Unknown/Other [*Narrative Box*]

*** Primary Tumor Size** (Note E)
Round to the nearest tenth of a centimeter.
__._ cm

*** Evidence of Extrathyroidal Extension of Primary Tumor on Imaging** (Note F)
Select single best answer.
__ No
__ Yes

*** Secondary Tumor Location** (Note D)
Select single best answer.
__ Right lobe
__ Left lobe
__ Isthmus
__ Pyramidal lobe
__ Unknown/Other [*Narrative Box*]

*** Secondary Tumor Size** (Note E)
Round to the nearest tenth of a centimeter.
___._ cm

*** Evidence of Extrathyroidal Extension of Secondary Tumor on Imaging** (Note F)
Select single best answer.
__ No
__ Yes

*** Additional Tumor Foci?**
Select single best answer.
__ No
__ Yes

[If "Yes" is selected, display the following:]
*** Tertiary Tumor Location** (Note D)
Select single best answer.
__ Right lobe
__ Left lobe
__ Isthmus
__ Pyramidal lobe
__ Unknown/Other [*Narrative Box*]

*** Tertiary Tumor Size** (Note E)
Round to the nearest tenth of a centimeter.
___._ cm

*** Evidence of Extrathyroidal Extension of Tertiary Tumor on Imaging** (Note F)
Select single best answer.
__ No
__ Yes

*** Preoperative Biopsy Performed** (Note G)
Select single best answer.
__ No
__ Yes
[If "Yes" is selected, display the following:]
*** Bethesda Category of Primary Tumor** (Note H)
Select single best answer.
__ I (Nondiagnostic)
__ II (Benign)
__ III (Atypia of unknown significance/follicular lesion of undetermined significance)
__ IV (Follicular neoplasm or suspicious for follicular neoplasm)
[If "IV" is selected, display the following:]
Hürthle Cell (Oncocytic) Type
Select single best answer.
__ No
__ Yes
__ Unknown or not specified

__ V (Suspicious for malignancy)
[If "V" is selected, display the following:]
Suspected Histology on FNA (Note I)
Select single best answer.
__ Suspicious for papillary carcinoma
__ Suspicious for medullary carcinoma
__ Suspicious for metastatic carcinoma
__ Suspicious for lymphoma
__ Unknown or not specified
__ VI (Malignant)
[If "VI" is selected, display the following:]
Suspected Histology on FNA (Note I)
Select single best answer.
__ Papillary thyroid carcinoma
__ Poorly differentiated carcinoma
__ Medullary thyroid carcinoma
__ Undifferentiated (anaplastic) thyroid carcinoma
__ Squamous-cell carcinoma
__ Carcinoma with mixed features—Specify [*Narrative Box*]
__ Unknown
__ Other—Describe [*Narrative Box*]

*** Molecular Testing Performed on Biopsy** (Note J)
Select single best answer.
__ Yes—Describe results [*Narrative Box*]
__ No

*** Clinical Nodal Status** (Note K)
Select all that apply.
__ No clinical evidence of lymph node metastases (cN0)
__ Imaging and/or clinical evidence of central compartment lymph node metastases (cN1a)
[If "cN1a" is selected, display the following:]
Select single best answer.
__ FNA performed
__ FNA not performed
__ Imaging and/or clinical evidence of lateral compartment lymph node metastases (cN1b)
[If "cN1b" is selected, display the following:]
Select single best answer.
__ FNA performed
__ FNA not performed
__ Imaging of lymph nodes was not performed

*** Procedure Performed** (Note L)
Select single best answer.
__ Thyroid lobectomy (right/left)
[If "Thyroid lobectomy" is selected, display the following:]
Select single best answer.
__ With isthmectomy
__ Without isthmectomy
__ Near-total thyroidectomy
__ Total thyroidectomy
__ Other [*Narrative Box*]

*** Intent of Surgery** (Note M)
Was the operation performed for curative intent? Select single best answer.
__ Yes
__ No
If no:
Select single best answer.
__ Diagnostic intent [*Narrative Box*]
__ Staging intent [*Narrative Box*]
__ Palliative intent [*Narrative Box*]

Intraoperative Findings

*** Macroscopic Disease Status of Primary Tumor** (Note N)
Select all that apply.
__ No evidence of gross extrathyroidal extension
__ Gross extrathyroidal extension of the primary tumor invading the strap muscles (T3b)
__ Gross extrathyroidal extension of the primary tumor invading subcutaneous soft tissue, larynx, trachea, esophagus, or recurrent laryngeal nerve (T4a)
[If "T4a" is selected, display the following:]
Select all that apply.
__ Soft tissue
__ Cricothyroid muscle
__ Larynx
__ Trachea
__ Esophagus
__ Recurrent laryngeal nerve
__ Other [*Narrative Box*]
__ Gross extrathyroidal extension of the primary tumor invading prevertebral fascia or encasing carotid artery or mediastinal vessels (T4b)
[If "T4b" is selected, display the following:]
Select all that apply.
__ Prevertebral fascia
__ Internal jugular vein
__ Carotid artery
__ Mediastinal vessels
__ Other [*Narrative Box*]

*** Central Compartment Lymph Node Dissection** (Note O)
Select single best answer.
__ Not performed
__ Prophylactic (N0)
[If "Prophylactic" is selected, display the following:]
Select single best answer.
__ Right
__ Left
__ Bilateral
__ Therapeutic (N1a)
[If "Therapeutic" is selected, display the following:]
Select single best answer.
__ Right
__ Left
__ Bilateral

Based on:
Select all that apply.
__ Preoperative imaging
__ Preoperative FNA
__ Visual examination
__ Intraoperative frozen section

*** Lateral Compartment Lymph Node Dissection** (Note P)
Select all that apply.
__ Not performed
__ Right
[If "Right" is selected, display the following:]
__ Level I
__ Level IIa __ Level IIb
__ Level III
__ Level IV
__ Level Va __ Level Vb
__ Left
[If "Left" is selected, display the following:]
__ Level I
__ Level IIa __ Level IIb
__ Level III
__ Level IV
__ Level Va __ Level Vb

*** Macroscopic Completeness of Resection** (Note Q)
At the conclusion of the case, was there evidence of gross disease? Select single best answer.
__ Macroscopic residual tumor at primary cancer site or regional nodal sites (R2 resection)—Describe where [*Narrative Box*]
__ No residual tumor (R0 resection)

Section 3: Additional Procedure Details (Note R)

Neuromonitoring Used (Note S)
Select single best answer.
__ No
__ Yes
[If "Yes" is selected, display the following:]
__ Nerve integrity confirmed at end of procedure
__ Nerve integrity not confirmed at end of procedure
[If "Nerve integrity not confirmed" is selected, display the following:]
__ Loss of signal
__ Not tested
__ Other (e.g., equipment failure) [*Narrative Box*]

Recurrent Laryngeal Nerve(s) (Note T)
Select single best answer for each category.
Right Recurrent Laryngeal Nerve
__ Not applicable
__ Anatomically intact, not involved with tumor
__ Involved with tumor
[If "Involved with tumor" is selected, display the following:]
__ Nerve resected en bloc with tumor
[If "Nerve resected" is selected, display the following:]
__ Nerve reconstructed [*Narrative Box*]
__ Nerve not reconstructed
__ Tumor shaved from nerve
__ Not seen
__ Other [*Narrative Box*]

Left Recurrent Laryngeal Nerve
__ Not applicable
__ Anatomically intact, not involved with tumor
__ Involved with tumor
[If "Involved with tumor" is selected, display the following:]
__ Nerve resected en bloc with tumor
[If "Nerve resected" is selected, display the following:]
__ Nerve reconstructed [*Narrative Box*]
__ Nerve not reconstructed
__ Tumor shaved from nerve
__ Not seen
__ Other [*Narrative Box*]

External Branch of the Superior Laryngeal Nerve(s) (Note U)
Select single best answer for each category.
Right EBSLN
__ Not applicable
__ Not seen
__ Anatomically intact, not involved with tumor
__ Involved with tumor

Left EBSLN
__ Not applicable
__ Not seen
__ Anatomically intact, not involved with tumor
__ Involved with tumor

Parathyroid Glands (Note V)
Select single best answer for each category.
Right Superior
__ Not applicable
__ Preserved in situ
__ Not identified
__ Autotransplanted [*Narrative Box*]

Right Inferior
__ Not applicable
__ Preserved in situ
__ Not identified
__ Autotransplanted [*Narrative Box*]

Left Superior
__ Not applicable
__ Preserved in situ
__ Not identified
__ Autotransplanted [*Narrative Box*]

Left Inferior
__ Not applicable
__ Preserved in situ
__ Not identified
__ Autotransplanted [*Narrative Box*]

Pyramidal Lobe (Note W)
Select single best answer.
__ Resected
__ Not resected
__ Not present

Operative Approach (Note X)
Select single best answer.
__ Open
__ Endoscopic
__ Other—Describe [*Narrative Box*]

Additional Surgical Information (Note Y)
Select single best answer.
__ No
__ Yes—Describe [*Narrative Box*]
__ Provided elsewhere [*Narrative Box*]

Intraoperative Complications (Note Z)
Select single best answer.
__ None
__ Yes—Describe [*Narrative Box*]

Synoptic Operative Report Summary Template (Mockup)

Thyroid Cancer

Patient Name: *[Autopopulate from EMR]*
Patient ID: *[Autopopulate from EMR]*
Date of Surgery: *[Autopopulate from EMR]*
Name of Surgeon: *[Autopopulate from EMR]*
Name of Co-Surgeon: *[Autopopulate from EMR]*
Name of Assistant(s): *[Autopopulate from EMR – Nurses notes]*
Indication for Surgery: *[Autopopulate from EMR;* ***or*** *override with EMR pick list]*
Preoperative Diagnosis: *[Autopopulate from EMR;* ***or*** *override with SOR selections]*
Postoperative Diagnosis: *[Autopopulate from EMR;* ***or*** *override with SOR selections]*
Procedure(s) Performed: *[Autopopulate from EMR;* ***or*** *override with SOR selections]*
Specimens Removed: *[Autopopulate from EMR – Nurses notes with override capability]*
Type of Anesthesia: *[Autopopulate from EMR – Anesthesia with override capability]*
Estimated Blood Loss: *[Autopopulate from EMR – Anesthesia with override capability]*
Drain/Implant *[Autopopulate from EMR – Nurses notes with override capability]*
Additional Administrative Details: *[Autopopulate from EMR;* ***or*** *Narrative text]*

Tumor-Specific Information
Clinical Staging (Preoperative)

[Fill from SOR: Number of Foci and, as applicable, Tumor Location, Tumor Size, and Evidence of Extrathyroidal Extension of Tumor on Imaging]
[Fill from SOR: Preoperative Biopsy Performed and, if applicable, Bethesda Category of Primary Tumor and, as applicable, Hürthle Cell (Oncocytic) Type or Suspected Histology on FNA]
[Fill from SOR: Molecular Testing Performed on Biopsy]
[Fill from SOR: Clinical Nodal Status]
[Fill from SOR: Procedure Performed]
[Fill from SOR: Intent of Surgery]

Intraoperative Findings

[Fill from SOR: Macroscopic Disease Status of Primary Tumor]
[Fill from SOR: Central Compartment Lymph Node Dissection]
[Fill from SOR: Lateral Compartment Lymph Node Dissection]
[Fill from SOR: Macroscopic Completeness of Resection]

Additional Procedure Details (Page 2)

[Fill from SOR: Neuromonitoring Used]
[Fill from SOR: Recurrent Laryngeal Nerve]
[Fill from SOR: External Branch of the Superior Laryngeal Nerve(s)]
[Fill from SOR: Parathyroid Glands]
[Fill from SOR: Pyramidal Lobe]
[Fill from SOR: Operative Approach]
[Fill from SOR: Additional Surgical Information]
[Fill from SOR: Intraoperative Complications]

Knowledge Platform

Introductory Comments:
This protocol is intended to standardize documentation and communication of critical components of thyroid cancer surgery. The following explanatory notes reference critical elements for cancer surgery as described in the *Operative Standards for Cancer Surgery*, Volume 2

Instructions

Each Explanatory Note is linked from a corresponding data element in the synoptic report above and contains additional materials and references that can be used to facilitate accurate completion of the report.

Section 1: EMR Autopopulated Information

Note A: EMR Autopopulated Information

Explanatory Comments: The following fields are intended to be prepopulated with site-specific identifiers and information from the EMR.

Patient Name
Patient ID
Date of Surgery
Name of Surgeon
Name of Co-Surgeon
Name of Assistant(s)
Indication for Surgery
Preoperative Diagnosis
Postoperative Diagnosis
Procedure(s) Performed
Specimens Removed
Type of Anesthesia
Estimated Blood Loss
Drain/Implant
Additional Administrative Details

The following table (Table 1) contains the initial FHIR mappings for data fields in section 1, which can be used to create auto-population functionality. Note that FHIR mappings may vary by site and electronic health record (EHR) and will be revised over time.

Table 1. Data Field FHIR Mappings – Thyroid Cancer *(Untested)*

SOR Fields	Resource Main Category	Mapping	Version 4.0	Filter Codes Type	Filter Codes	Resource Link	Additional Links
Patient Name	Individual	patient.name	R4			https://fhir.cerner.com/millennium/r4/individuals/patient/	
MRN	Individual	patient.id	R4			https://fhir.cerner.com/millennium/r4/individuals/patient/	
Date of Surgery	Procedure	Procedure.performed[x]	R4	dateTime|Period|string|Age|Range	N/A	https://hl7.org/fhir/R4/procedure-definitions.html#Procedure.encounter	See Choice of Data Types for further information about how [x] is used
Name of Surgeon	Scheduling	Appointment.participant.required	R4	SNOMED	1421009-766788081000087100	http://hl7.org/fhir/R4/appointment-definitions.html#Appointment.participant.actor	
Name of Co-Surgeon	Scheduling	Appointment.participant.required	R4	SNOMED	1421009-766788081000087100	http://hl7.org/fhir/R4/appointment-definitions.html#Appointment.participant.actor	
Name of Assistant(s)	Scheduling	Appointment.participant.required	R4	SNOMED	1421009-766788081000087100	http://hl7.org/fhir/R4/appointment-definitions.html#Appointment.participant.actor	
Indication for Surgery	Procedure	Procedure.reasoncode	R4	ICD10	C73	http://hl7.org/fhir/procedure-definitions.html#Procedure.reasonCode	
Preoperative Diagnosis (ICD10)	Condition	Condition.Code	R4	ICD10	C73	https://hl7.org/fhir/r4/condition-definitions.html#Condition.code	https://hl7.org/fhir/r4/valueset-condition-code.html
Postoperative Diagnosis (ICD10)	Condition	Condition.Code	R4	ICD10	C73	https://hl7.org/fhir/r4/condition-definitions.html#Condition.code	
Procedure Performed	Procedure	Procedure.Code	R4	ICD10	0G2,0G5, 0G8, 0G9, 0GB, 0GC 0GH, 0GJ 0GM, 0GN 0GP, 0GQ 0GS, 0GT 0GW	https://hl7.org/fhir/R4/valueset-procedure-code.html	
Specimens Removed	Observation Procedure	Observation.specimen DiagnosticReport.specimen	R4	ICD 10 Procedure	0GPK	https://hl7.org/fhir/R4/procedure-definitions.html#Procedure.reasonReference	https://hl7.org/fhir/R4/observation-definitions.html#Observation.value_x_

Type of Anesthesia	Diagnostic	Observation.code	R4	LOINC	10213-7	https://hl7.org/fhir/R4/valueset-observation-codes.html	
Estimated Blood Loss	Diagnostic	Observation.value	R4	LOINC	59770-8	https://hl7.org/fhir/R4/observation-definitions.html#Observation.value_x_	
Drain/Implant	Procedure	Procedure.focalDevice	R4	ICD 10 Procedure	0G9G 0G9H 0G9K	https://hl7.org/fhir/R4/observation-definitions.html#Observation.value_x_	
Additional Administrative Details	N/A	N/A					
Surgery Location (hidden field)	Procedure	Encounter.location				https://hl7.org/fhir/r4/encounter-definitions.html#Encounter.location	

Section 2: Tumor-Specific Information

Note B: Tumor-Specific Information

Explanatory Comments: This section of the synoptic operative report contains critical oncology data elements supported by evidence and best practice, as well as data fields defined by the STORE manual and submitted to hospital registries for NCDB and state registry reporting. There are data fields in this section related to findings and/or treatments in both the preoperative and intraoperative phases of care. To complete the preoperative data fields assumes that the patient has undergone comprehensive assessment which may include/includes physical examination, radiologic assessment, fine needle aspiration (FNA) biopsy, and/or molecular testing. For additional details, please refer to the *Operative Standards for Cancer Surgery,* Volume 2, pages 2–12.

Note C: Number of Foci

Explanatory Comments: Tumors to be included when making the decision between unifocal and multifocal are those that: a) have been biopsied and/or b) are dominant lesion(s) for which the surgery is being performed. These tumors include all benign, indeterminate, and malignant nodules that meet either of these criteria.

Note D: Tumor Location

Explanatory Comments: Tumor location should be recorded for each focus that: a) has been biopsied and/or b) are dominant lesion(s) for which the surgery is being performed. Choose the option that best describes the location. Only when the tumor is unable to be categorized into other options should the “Unknown/Other” selection be made, and detail should be included in the narrative box as to why this selection was chosen. For multifocal disease, fields are provided to record tumor location for up to three tumors.

Note E: Tumor Size

Explanatory Comments: For each foci whose location was detailed, provide the single largest diameter in centimeters, rounding to the nearest tenth of a centimeter.

Note F: Evidence of Extrathyroidal Extension of Tumor on Imaging

Explanatory Comments: According to the AJCC, "Extrathyroidal extension refers to the involvement of perithyroidal soft tissues by direct extension from the thyroid primary. Invasion outside the thyroid that can be identified *by imaging* or intraoperative findings ranges from T3b disease (gross extrathyroidal extension involving only strap muscles) to T4a disease (demonstrating gross extrathyroidal extension invading the subcutaneous soft tissues, larynx, trachea, esophagus, muscle, or recurrent laryngeal nerve) to T4b disease (demonstrating gross extrathyroidal extension invading the prevertebral fascia or encasing the carotid artery or mediastinal vessels)." If there is evidence supportive of the above described extrathyroidal extension on any imaging studies performed (ultrasound, CT, and/or MRI), select "yes". If the findings are inconclusive or negative for extrathyroidal extension, select "no." For multifocal disease, fields are provided to record this information for up to three tumors. For additional details, please refer to the *Operative Standards for Cancer Surgery*, Volume 2, pages 8–11 and the *AJCC Cancer Staging Manual, Eighth Edition*, Chapter 73 (Thyroid – Differentiated and Anaplastic Thyroid Cancer) and Chapter 74 (Thyroid – Medullary).

Note G: Preoperative Biopsy Performed

Explanatory Comments: If a fine needle aspiration (FNA) or core needle biopsy (CNB) was performed on the thyroid nodule(s) prior to the index surgical procedure, indicate yes or no accordingly.

Note H: Bethesda Category of Primary Tumor

Explanatory Comments: The Bethesda System for Reporting Thyroid Cytopathology (TBSRTC) has established a standardized, category-based reporting system for thyroid FNA specimens. Every thyroid FNA report should begin with one of six diagnostic categories:

(I) nondiagnostic or unsatisfactory;
(II) benign;
(III) atypia of undetermined significance (AUS) or follicular lesion of undetermined significance (FLUS);
(IV) follicular neoplasm or suspicious for a follicular neoplasm;
(V) suspicious for malignancy; and
(VI) malignant.

There is a choice of two different names for some of the categories. Laboratories are to choose the one they prefer and use it exclusively for that category. Each category has an implied cancer risk that ranges from 0% to 3% for benign to nearly 100% for the malignant category. If category IV, specify whether Hürthle cell (oncocytic) type, if known. For additional details, please refer to the 2017 Bethesda System for Reporting Thyroid Cytopathology.

Note I: Suspected Histology on FNA

Explanatory Comments: Thyroid cancer comprises several distinct histologies arising from thyroid follicular or parafollicular C cells. Papillary thyroid cancers and follicular thyroid cancers (and their respective variants) are classified as differentiated thyroid cancers that arise from thyroid follicular cells and in general have excellent prognosis, with 10-year survival of 90–95%. Poorly differentiated thyroid cancers probably arise from either PTCs or FTCs and have a poorer prognosis, with 10-year survival rates approximating 50%. Conversely, anaplastic thyroid carcinoma is an aggressive undifferentiated tumor of thyroid follicular cell origin and, in most series, is associated with 5-year survival rates of less than 10%. The "Other" category should be used for metastatic carcinoma, non-Hodgkin lymphoma, and other suspected histologies not listed. For additional details, please refer to the *AJCC Cancer Staging Manual, Eighth Edition,* Chapter 73 (Thyroid – Differentiated and Anaplastic Thyroid Cancer) and Chapter 74 (Thyroid – Medullary).

Note J: Molecular Testing Performed on Biopsy

Explanatory Comments: If preoperative evaluation included molecular testing from an FNA or core biopsy specimen, indicate yes or no accordingly and describe results as needed. The specific type of test is not required.

Note K: Clinical Nodal Status

Explanatory Comments: This field seeks to document data on clinical evidence, either by physical exam or imaging, of cervical nodal metastases before surgery. The type of imaging is not specified and could be any appropriate study. If imaging was performed and there was no evidence of nodal disease, the patient would be considered cN0. If there is evidence of nodal disease in the central or lateral compartments, the patient would be considered either cN1a or cN1b respectively. If no imaging was performed, indicate as such. Furthermore, if there is evidence of N1a or N1b disease, the information about preoperative FNA is requested. Physical exam does not suffice to define the patient as cN0 but could qualify the patient a cN1.

Table 3. AJCC Definitions of Regional Lymph Node (N) for Thyroid

N Category	N Criteria
cNX	Regional lymph nodes cannot be assessed
cN0	No evidence of locoregional lymph node metastasis
cN0a	One or more cytologically or histologically confirmed benign lymph nodes
cN0b	No radiologic or clinical evidence of locoregional lymph node metastasis
cN1	Metastasis to regional nodes
cN1a	Metastasis to level VI or VII (pretracheal, paratracheal, or prelaryngeal/Delphian, or upper mediastinal) lymph nodes. This can be unilateral or bilateral disease.
cN1b	Metastasis to unilateral, bilateral, or contralateral lateral neck lymph nodes (levels I, II, III, IV, or V) or retropharyngeal lymph nodes

AJCC Cancer Staging Manual, Eighth Edition, Chapter 73 (Thyroid – Differentiated and Anaplastic Thyroid Cancer) and Chapter 74 (Thyroid – Medullary)

Note L: Procedure Performed

Explanatory Comments: Extent of surgical treatment needs to be clearly described. This field allows four choices. The selection for thyroid lobectomy (either left or right) includes total and near-total thyroid lobectomy procedures and should be documented as either with or without isthmectomy. Near-total thyroidectomy should be chosen when a near-total or subtotal thyroidectomy was performed. Total thyroidectomy should be chosen when a total bilobar resection was performed. Nodulectomy, isthmectomy, and open biopsy are not common procedures for thyroid cancer but would fall under the “other” category if performed and may be described using the narrative box, along with any other procedures not listed.

NCDB coding instructions for *Rx Summ–Surg 2023* [1291] are detailed in the STORE 2023 manual. Site-specific surgery codes for the thyroid gland can be found in Appendix A and those relevant to this synoptic operative report are summarized below in Table 4.

Table 4. Relevant NCDB Site-Specific Surgery Codes for Thyroid Gland Adapted from STORE Manual

NCDB Code	Definition
A200	Lobectomy and/or isthmectomy
A210	Lobectomy ONLY
A220	Isthmectomy ONLY
A230	Lobectomy WITH isthmus
A300	Removal of a lobe and partial removal of the contralateral lobe
A400	Subtotal or near total thyroidectomy
A500	Total thyroidectomy
A800	Thyroidectomy, NOS

ACS Standards for Oncology Registry Entry (STORE) 2023. Appendix A: Site-Specific Surgery Codes, Thyroid Gland.
*This table does not include codes A250, A260, and A270 which fall outside the scope of this protocol.

Note M: Intent of Surgery

Explanatory Comments: Intent should be assigned postoperatively by the operating surgeon on the basis of preoperative evaluation and intraoperative management and should be documented as part of the operative report. Curative operations generally include complete resection of the primary tumor and regional lymphadenectomy for therapeutic or staging purposes. If the operation was not performed for curative intent, response options are provided for diagnostic, staging, or palliative intent along with narrative boxes to record any additional information.

For some cancers, a surgical procedure such as a thyroid lobectomy or a lymph node dissection is required for diagnostic purposes. When the goal is to completely resect the cancer along with any extrathyroidal cervical disease, the operative intent is curative. If the operation was performed for bleeding or symptoms from compression or invasion, but the goal was not a curative resection, it should be indicated as palliative.

Note N: Macroscopic Disease Status of Primary Tumor

Explanatory Comments: In the context of intraoperative findings in this protocol for cancer surgery documentation, TNM categories from the American Joint Committee on Cancer (AJCC) are not designated with clinical (lower case "c" prefix) nor pathological (lower case "p" prefix) classifications. Determination of pathological classification involves a synthesis of information from multiple sources including clinical staging, operative findings, and pathological evaluation of resected surgical specimen(s). Complete information on TNM categories, clinical/pathological classifications, and the overall process of cancer staging can be found in the *AJCC Cancer Staging Manual, Eighth Edition*.

Extrathyroidal extension refers to involvement of the perithyroidal soft tissue by direct extension of the thyroid primary. The operative report should document extrathyroidal extension when present to assure appropriate T staging of the tumor. Gross extrathyroidal extension in differentiated thyroid cancers increases disease persistence/recurrence and decreases survival. For additional details, please refer to the *Operative Standards for Cancer Surgery*, Volume 2, pages 19–22.

Note O: Central Compartment Lymph Node Dissection

Explanatory Comments: In the context of intraoperative findings in this protocol for cancer surgery documentation, TNM categories from the American Joint Committee on Cancer (AJCC) are not designated with clinical (lower case "c" prefix) nor pathological (lower case "p" prefix) classifications. Determination of pathological classification involves a synthesis of information from multiple sources including clinical staging, operative findings, and pathological evaluation of resected surgical specimen(s). Complete information on TNM categories, clinical/pathological classifications, and the overall process of cancer staging can be found in the *AJCC Cancer Staging Manual, Eighth Edition*.

Central compartment lymph node dissection for thyroid cancer constitutes removal of lymph nodes in central neck. The term "central neck" refers to level VI and VII (superior mediastinum), as shown in Figure 1 below. Gross inspection of the central compartment lymph tissue should be performed at the time of the thyroidectomy. Nodal dissection in the central compartment should be performed en-bloc within the anatomic boundaries of the hyoid bone cranially, the innominate artery caudally on the right and the corresponding axial plane caudally on the left, the common carotid arteries laterally, the deep layer of the cervical fascia posteriorly, and the superficial layer of the cervical fascio anteriorly, to include the thyroid and parathyroid glands, the level VI lymph nodes, the upper portion of the level VII lymph nodes, and the cervical portion of the thymus. The surgeon should document the extent of the dissection: ipsilateral or bilateral central compartment dissection. Regional lymph node metastases appear to have strong prognostic significance in most differentiated thyroid cancers. For additional details, please refer to the *Operative Standards for Cancer Surgery*, Volume 2, pages 29–32 and the *AJCC Cancer Staging Manual, Eighth Edition,* Chapter 73 (Thyroid – Differentiated and Anaplastic Thyroid Cancer) and Chapter 74 (Thyroid – Medullary).

NCDB coding instructions for *Scope of Regional Lymph Node Surgery* [1292], used to identify the removal, biopsy, or aspiration of regional lymph node(s) at the time of surgery of the primary site or during a separate surgical event, are detailed in the STORE 2023 manual. NCDB coding instructions for *Scope of Regional Lymph Node Surgery at this Facility* [672] are also detailed on in the STORE 2023 manual.

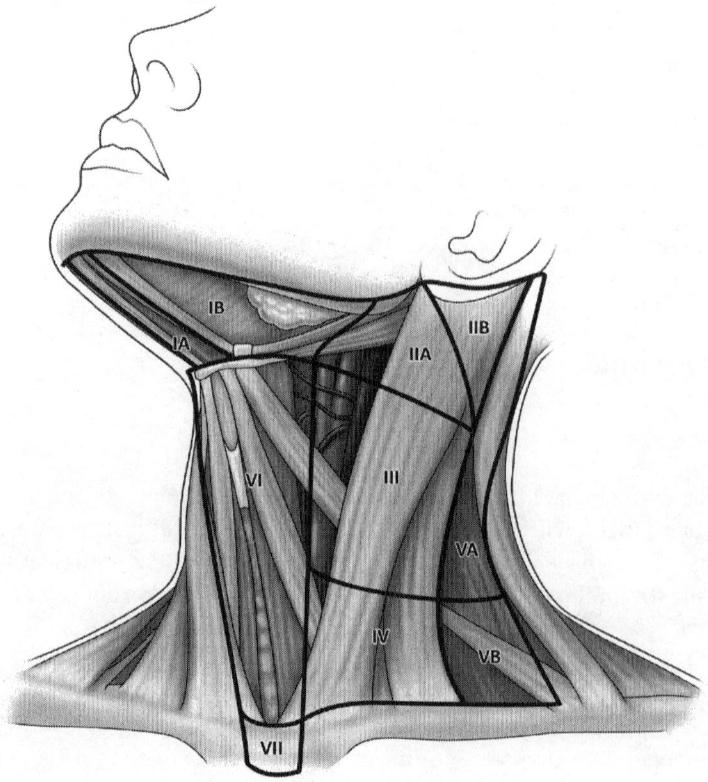

Figure 1. Nodal basin levels of the neck.

Note P: Lateral Compartment Lymph Node Dissection

Explanatory Comments: Lateral compartment lymph node dissection refers to removal of nodes in Levels I, II, III, IV, and V, as shown in Figure 1 in Note P. Lateral neck regional node disease carries a worse prognosis than central neck regional disease. Several studies have demonstrated that lateral neck lymph node metastasis is associated with compromised survival. Levels IIA, III, IV, and VB should be included routinely in a lateral compartment neck dissection for metastatic papillary thyroid carcinoma. Levels I, IIB, and VA should be included based on the burden of disease in adjacent compartments or if there is clinical evidence of disease at the time of surgery. For additional details and anatomic landmarks of each nodal basin level, please refer to the *Operative Standards for Cancer Surgery*, Volume 2, pages 38–43.

NCDB coding instructions for *Scope of Regional Lymph Node Surgery* [1292], used to identify the removal, biopsy, or aspiration of regional lymph node(s) at the time of surgery of the primary site or during a separate surgical event, are detailed in the STORE 2023 manual. NCDB coding instructions for *Scope of Regional Lymph Node Surgery at this Facility* [672] are also detailed on in the STORE 2023 manual.

Note Q: Macroscopic Completeness of Resection

Explanatory Comments: The operative report must document any findings of gross residual disease at the end of the case. Definitions for R Designation from the AJCC are summarized below in Table 5.

Patients with a grossly positive margin (R2 or incomplete resection) have a statistically higher risk of recurrence and disease specific death. For additional details, please refer to the *Operative Standards for Cancer Surgery*, Volume 2, pages 19–22, and the *AJCC Cancer Staging Manual, Eighth Edition,* Chapter 1 (Principles of Cancer Staging).

Table 5. Definition of R Designation (Residual Tumor After Treatment)

R	R Definition
RX	Presence of residual tumor cannot be assessed
R0	No residual tumor
R1	Microscopic residual tumor
R2	Macroscopic residual tumor at the primary cancer site or regional nodal sites (This designation is not used to indicate metastatic disease identified but not resected at surgical exploration.)

AJCC Cancer Staging Manual, Eighth Edition, Chapter 1 (Principles of Cancer Staging).

Section 3: Additional Procedure Details

Note R: Additional Procedure Details

Explanatory Comments: The following fields have been included for the synoptic operative report to represent a complete record of information so that it will not only fulfill surgeon and institutional documentation needs, but also can fulfill regulatory requirements. The inclusion of open-text narrative fields provides sufficient flexibility for all aspects of surgical care to be recorded and for multiple functions, such as registry submission and generation of billing codes, to be permissible.

Note S: Neuromonitoring Used

Explanatory Comments: Intraoperative monitoring of the recurrent laryngeal nerve(s) and the external branch of the superior laryngeal nerve(s) may be utilized as an intraoperative adjunct for identification and confirmation of the functionality of the nerve. There are no level 1 data to support the use of nerve monitoring in reducing the risk of injury to the recurrent laryngeal nerves. For additional details, please refer to the *Operative Standards for Cancer Surgery,* Volume 2, page 18.

Note T: Recurrent Laryngeal Nerve(s)

Explanatory Comments: The recurrent laryngeal nerve should be identified and preserved during thyroidectomy. The nerve is most reliably identified at the point where it emerges from the mediastinum, at the tubercle of Zuckerkandl, and/or at the insertion point into the larynx. A thyroid surgeon should have a comprehensive understanding of the anatomy of the nerves, including both normal and variants. For additional details, please refer to the *Operative Standards for Cancer Surgery,* Volume 2, pages 17–18.

Note U: External Branch of the Superior Laryngeal Nerve(s)

Explanatory Comments: The external branch of the superior laryngeal nerve may be identified during thyroidectomy and can be documented here. To avoid injury, the superior pole of the thyroid should be dissected near the thyroid capsule and away from the muscle of the cricothyroid.

Note V: Parathyroid Glands

Explanatory Comments: During thyroidectomy, the surgeon should attempt to identify and preserve the parathyroid glands to minimize the risk of both transient and permanent hypoparathyroidism. The location of the glands may be variable. Nonviable parathyroid glands should be autotransplanted, although the site of autotransplantation may vary, based on surgeon preference. Prior to autotransplantation, pathologic confirmation should be obtained. Details can be documented for the right superior, right inferior, left superior, and left inferior glands. For additional details, please refer to the *Operative Standards for Cancer Surgery*, Volume 2, pages 13–17.

Note W: Pyramidal Lobe

Explanatory Comments: This data field can be used to indicate whether the pyramidal lobe was resected, not resected, or not present. If present, the pyramidal lobe of the thyroid should be identified and resected to minimize the likelihood of recurrent disease at this site.

Note X: Operative Approach

Explanatory Comments: This data field can be used to document the surgical approach used for the operation, which may be needed for certain billing and coding requirements.

NCDB codes are provided below in Table 6 for the *Approach – Surgery of the Primary Site at this Facility (RxHospSurgApp 2010)* [668] data item from STORE 2023.

Table 6. NCDB Codes for *Approach – Surgery of the Primary Site at this Facility* from STORE Manual

NCDB Code	Label
0	No surgical procedure of primary site at this facility; Diagnosed at autopsy
1	Robotic assisted
2	Robotic converted to open
3	Minimally invasive (such as endoscopic or laparoscopic)
4	Minimally invasive (endoscopic or laparoscopic) converted to open
5	Open or approach unspecified

ACS Standards for Oncology Registry Entry (STORE) 2023. Approach – Surgery of the Primary Site at this Facility (RxHospSurgApp 2010).
*This table has been amended to remove code 9 (Unknown whether the surgery was performed at this facility) as it would not be an appropriate code in the context of this report.

Note Y: Additional Surgical Information

Explanatory Comments: While concordance with operative standards has been the primary focus of this synoptic operative report, end user focus groups requested the scope of the tool to be expanded in order for it to comply with all surgical reporting requirements. As a result, this report can now be considered a comprehensive operative report and it can be used to help generate billing codes and output data into hospital registries.

There was not sufficient consensus, however, on non-cancer surgical information, such as patient positioning, incision location, and techniques for closure, so narrative text options are provided for inserting information you consider important.

Note Z: Intraoperative Complications

Explanatory Comments: Intraoperative complications are rare, but it is still important to document them regardless of whether they are related to focal surgical difficulties or systemic events that may relate to patient positioning, delivery of anesthesia, or other aspects of the surgical procedure.

References

1. Amin MB, Edge SB, Greene FL, et al, eds. *AJCC Cancer Staging Manual*. 8th ed. New York, NY: Springer; 2017.
2. Cibas ES and Ali SZ. The 2017 Bethesda System for Reporting Thyroid Cytopathology. *Thyroid*. 2017;27(11):1341–1346.
3. Commission on Cancer. *Standards for Oncology Registry Entry (STORE)*. Chicago, IL: American College of Surgeons; 2023.
4. Katz MH, American College of Surgeons Clinical Research Program. *Operative Standards for Cancer Surgery*. Vol 2. Chicago, IL: Wolters Kluwer; 2018.

Made in the USA
Monee, IL
07 May 2026

49714981R00015